Vegan Keto Cookbook

Mouth-Watering Vegan-Friendly Recipes to Save Time & Money!

Arooj Leonard

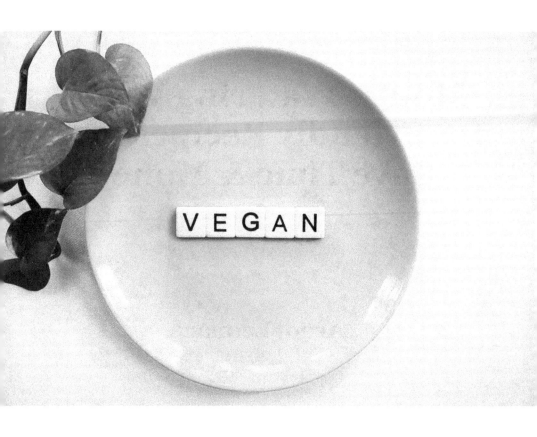

CONTENTS

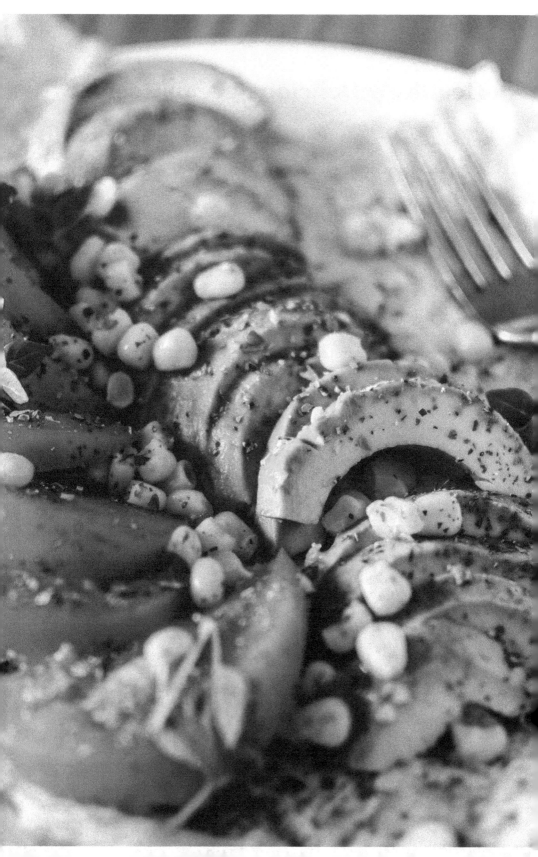

Healthy & Delicious Vegan Recipes

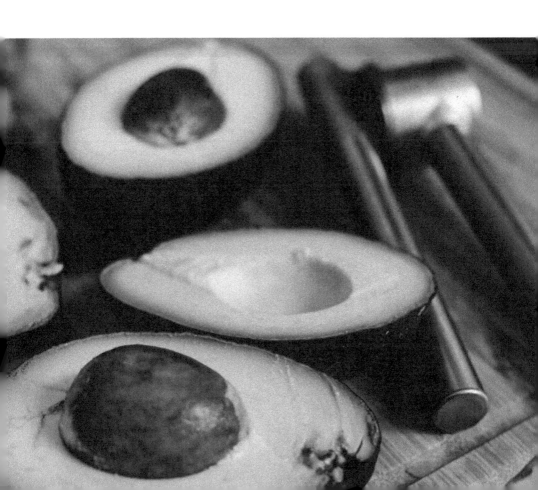

Sauteed Spinach with Spicy Tofu

Ingredients for 4 servings

2 tbsp olive oil

14 oz block tofu, pressed and cubed

1 celery stalk, chopped

1 bunch scallions, chopped

1 tsp cayenne pepper

1 tsp garlic powder

2 tbsp Worcestershire sauce

Salt and black pepper, to taste

1 lb spinach, chopped

½ tsp turmeric powder

¼ tsp dried basil

Directions and Total Time: approx. 25 minutes

In a large skillet over medium heat, warm 1 tablespoon of olive oil.

Stir in tofu cubes and cook for 8 minutes.

Place in scallions and celery; cook for 5 minutes until soft.

Stir in cayenne, Worcestershire sauce, black pepper, salt, and garlic; cook

for 3 more minutes; set aside.

In the same pan, warm the remaining 1 tablespoon of oil.

Add in spinach and the remaining seasonings and cook for 4 minutes.

Mix in tofu mixture and serve warm.

Per serving: Cal 205; Fat 12.5g; Net Carbs 7.6g; Protein 7.7g

Poppy Seed Coleslaw

Ingredients for 4 servings

Dressing

2 tbsp olive oil

1 cup poppy seeds

2 cups water

2 tbsp green onions, chopped

1 garlic clove, minced

1 lime, freshly squeezed

Salt and black pepper, to taste

¼ tsp dill, minced

1 tbsp yellow mustard

Salad

½ head white cabbage, shredded

1 carrot, shredded

1 shallot, sliced

2 tbsp Kalamata olives, pitted

Directions and Total Time: approx. 3 hours and 15 minutes

In a food processor, place olive oil, water, green onion, mustard, dill, lime

juice, salt, and black pepper to taste.

Pulse until well incorporated.

Add in poppy seeds and mix well.

Place cabbage, carrot, and onion in a bowl and mix to combine.

Transfer to a salad plate, pour the dressing over and top with kalamata

olives to serve.

Per serving: Cal 235; Fat 17.3g; Net Carbs 6.4g; Protein 8.1g

Vegetable Stew

Ingredients for 4 servings

2 tbsp olive oil

1 turnip, chopped

1 onion, chopped

2 garlic cloves, pressed

½ cup celery, chopped

1 carrot, chopped

1 cup wild mushrooms, sliced

2 tbsp dry white wine

2 tbsp rosemary, chopped

1 thyme sprig, chopped

4 cups vegetable stock

½ tsp chili pepper

1 tsp smoked paprika

2 tomatoes, chopped

1 tbsp flax seed meal

Directions and Total Time: approx. 25 minutes

Cook onion, carrot, celery, mushrooms, paprika, chili pepper, and garlic in

warm oil over medium heat for 5-6 minutes until tender; set the vegetables

aside.

Stir in wine to deglaze the stockpot's bottom.

Place in thyme and rosemary.

Pour in tomatoes, vegetable stock, reserved vegetables and turnip and

allow to boil.

On low heat, allow the mixture to simmer for 15 minutes while covered.

Stir in flax seed meal to thicken the stew.

Plate into individual bowls and serve.

Per serving: Cal 164; Fat 11.3g; Net Carbs 8.2g; Protein 3.3g

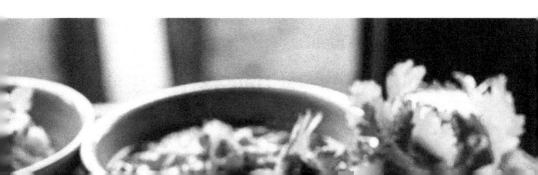

Basil Tofu with Cashew Nuts

Ingredients for 4 servings

3 tsp olive oil

1 cup extra firm tofu, cubed

¼ cup cashew nuts

1 ½ tbsp coconut aminos

3 tbsp vegetable broth

1 garlic clove, minced

1 tsp cayenne pepper

½ tsp turmeric powder

Salt and black pepper, to taste

2 tsp sunflower seeds

10 basil leaves, torn

1 tbsp balsamic vinegar

Directions and Total Time: approx. 13 minutes

Warm olive oil in a frying pan over medium heat.

Add in tofu and fry until golden, turning once, for about 6 minutes.

Pour in the cashew nuts and cook for 2 minutes.

Stir in the remaining ingredients except for the balsamic vinegar and basil,

set heat to medium-low and cook for 5 more minutes.

Drizzle with the balsamic vinegar, season to taste, sprinkle with basil and

serve.

Per serving: Cal 245; Fat 19g; Net Carbs 5.5g; Protein 12g

Avocado Boats

Ingredients for 4 servings

2 avocados, halved and stoned

1 tomato, chopped

1 cucumber, chopped

¼ cup walnuts, ground

2 carrots, chopped

1 garlic clove

1 tsp lemon juice

1 tbsp soy sauce

Salt and black pepper, to taste

Directions and Total Time: approx. 10 minutes

To make the filling, in a mixing bowl, mix soy sauce, tomato, carrots,

avocado pulp, cucumber, lemon juice, walnuts, and garlic.

Add black pepper and salt.

Plate the mixture into the avocado halves.

Scatter walnuts over to serve.

Per serving: Cal 272; Fat 25g; Net Carbs 6.1g;
Protein 4g

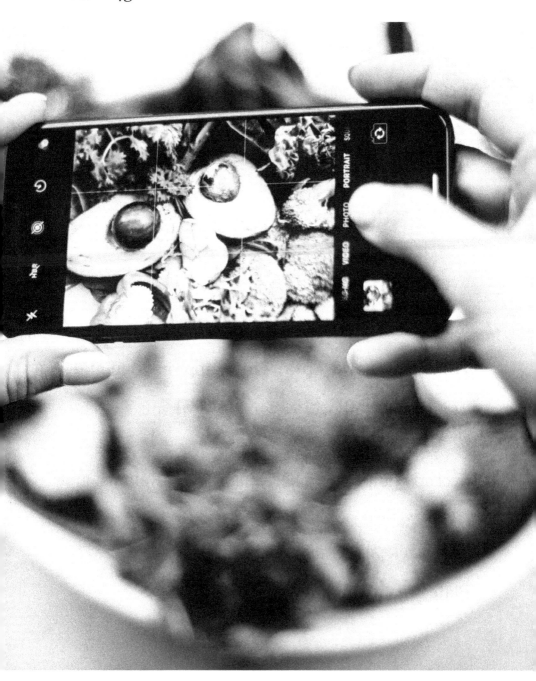

Fennel & Celeriac with Chili Tomato Sauce

Ingredients for 4 servings

2 tbsp olive oil

1 garlic clove, crushed

½ celeriac, sliced

½ fennel bulb, sliced

¼ cup vegetable stock

Sea salt and black pepper, to taste

Sauce

2 tomatoes, halved

2 tbsp olive oil

½ cup onions, chopped

2 cloves garlic, minced

1 chili, minced

1 bunch fresh basil, chopped

1 tbsp fresh cilantro, chopped

Salt and black pepper, to taste

Directions and Total Time: approx. 20 minutes

Set a pan over medium-high heat and warm olive oil.

Add in garlic and sauté for 1 minute.

Stir in celeriac and fennel slices, stock and cook until softened.

Sprinkle with black pepper and salt.

Brush olive oil to the tomato halves.

Microwave for 15 minutes; get rid of any excess liquid.

Remove the cooked tomatoes to a food processor; add the rest of the

Ingredients for the sauce and puree to obtain the desired consistency.

Serve the celeriac and fennel topped with tomato sauce.

Per serving: Cal 145; Fat 15g; Net Carbs 5.3g; Protein 2.1g

Tofu & Hazelnut Loaded Zucchini

Ingredients for 4 servings

2 tbsp olive oil

12 oz firm tofu, drained and crumbled

2 garlic cloves, pressed

½ cup onions, chopped

2 cups crushed tomatoes

¼ tsp dried oregano

Salt and black pepper to taste

¼ tsp chili pepper

2 zucchinis, cut into halves, scoop out the insides

¼ cup hazelnuts, chopped

2 tbsp cilantro, chopped

Directions and Total Time: approx. 50 minutes

Sauté onion, garlic, and tofu in olive oil for 5 minutes until softened.

Place in scooped zucchini flesh, 1 cup of tomatoes, oregano, and chili pepper.

Season with salt, and pepper and cook for 6 minutes.

Preheat oven to 390 F.

Pour the remaining tomatoes in a baking dish.

Spoon the tofu mixture into the zucchini shells.

Arrange the zucchini boats in the baking dish.

Bake for about 30 minutes.

Sprinkle with hazelnuts and continue baking for 5 to 6 more minutes.

Scatter with cilantro to serve.

Per serving: Cal 234; Fat 18.3g; Net Carbs 5.9g; Protein 12.5g

One-Pot Ratatouille with Pecans

Ingredients for 4 servings

2 tbsp olive oil

1 eggplant, sliced

1 zucchini, sliced

1 red onion, sliced

14 oz canned tomatoes

1 red bell peppers, sliced

1 yellow bell pepper, sliced

1 cloves garlic, sliced

¼ cup basil leaves, chop half

2 sprigs thyme

1 tbsp balsamic vinegar

½ lemon, zested

¼ cup pecans, chopped

Salt and black pepper to taste

Directions and Total Time: approx. 47 minutes

Place a casserole pot over medium heat and warm the olive oil.

Sauté the eggplants, zucchinis, and bell peppers for 5 minutes.

Spoon the veggies into a large bowl.

In the same pan, sauté garlic, onion, and thyme leaves for 5 minutes and

return the cooked veggies to the pan along with the canned tomatoes,

balsamic vinegar, chopped basil, salt, and pepper to taste.

Stir and cover the pot, and cook the ingredients on low heat for 30 minutes.

Stir in the remaining basil leaves, lemon zest, and adjust the seasoning to

serve.

Per serving: Cal 188; Fat 13g; Net Carbs 8.3g; Protein 4.5g

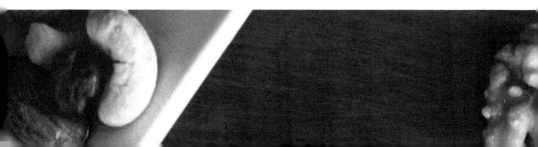

Parsnip & Carrot Strips with Walnut Sauce

Ingredients for 4 servings

2 tbsp olive oil

2 carrots, cut into strips

2 parsnips, cut into strips

½ cup water

Salt and black pepper to taste

1 tsp rosemary, chopped

Walnut sauce

½ cup walnuts

3 tbsp nutritional yeast

Salt and black pepper, to taste

¼ tsp onion powder

½ tsp garlic powder

¼ cup olive oil

Directions and Total Time: approx. 15 minutes

Set a pan over medium heat and warm oil; cook the parsnips and carrots

for 1 minute as you stir.

Add in water and cook for an additional 6 minutes.

Sprinkle with rosemary, salt, and pepper; transfer to a serving platter.

Place all sauce ingredients in a food processor and pulse until you attain

the required consistency.

Pour the sauce over the vegetables and serve.

Per serving: Cal 338; Fat 28.6g; Net Carbs 9.7g; Protein 6.5g

Pumpkin & Bell Pepper Noodles with Avocado Sauce

Ingredients for 4 servings

½ lb pumpkin, spiralized

½ lb bell peppers, spiralized

2 tbsp olive oil

2 avocados, chopped

1 lemon, juiced and zested

2 tbsp sesame oil

2 tbsp cilantro, chopped

1 onion, chopped

1 jalapeño pepper, deveined and minced

Salt and black pepper, to taste

2 tbsp pumpkin seeds

Directions and Total Time: approx. 15 minutes

Toast the pumpkin seeds in a dry nonstick skillet, stirring frequently for a

minute until golden; set aside.

Add in oil and sauté bell peppers and pumpkin for 8 minutes.

Remove to a serving platter.

Combine avocados, sesame oil, onion, jalapeño pepper, lemon juice, and

lemon zest in a food processor and pulse to obtain a creamy mixture.

Adjust the seasoning and pour over the vegetable noodles, top with the

pumpkin seeds and serve.

Per serving: Cal 673; Fat 59g; Net Carbs 9.8g; Protein 22.9g

Oven-Roasted Asparagus with Romesco Sauce

Ingredients for 4 servings

1 lb asparagus spears, trimmed

2 tbsp olive oil

Salt and black pepper, to taste

½ tsp paprika

Romesco sauce

2 red bell peppers, roasted

2 tsp olive oil

2 tbsp almond flour

½ cup scallions, chopped

1 garlic clove, minced

1 tbsp lemon juice

½ tsp chili pepper

Salt and black pepper, to taste

2 tbsp rosemary, chopped

Directions and Total Time: approx. 15 minutes

In a food processor, pulse together the bell peppers, salt, black pepper,

garlic, lemon juice, scallions, almond flour, 2 tsp of olive oil and chili pepper.

Mix evenly and set aside.

Preheat oven to 390 F and line a baking sheet with parchment paper.

Add asparagus spears to the baking sheet.

Toss with 2 tbsp of olive oil, paprika, black pepper, and salt.

Bake until cooked through for 9 minutes.

Transfer to a serving plate, pour the sauce over and

Tofu & Vegetable Casserole

Ingredients for 4 servings

10 oz tofu, pressed and cubed

2 tsp olive oil

1 cup leeks, chopped

1 garlic clove, minced

½ cup celery, chopped

½ cup carrot, chopped

1 ½ lb Brussels sprouts, shredded

1 habanero pepper, chopped

2 ½ cups mushrooms, sliced

1 ½ cups vegetable stock

2 tomatoes, chopped

2 thyme sprigs, chopped

1 rosemary sprig, chopped

2 bay leaves

Salt and ground black pepper to taste

Directions and Total Time: approx. 45 minutes

Set a pot over medium heat and warm oil.

Add in garlic and leeks and sauté until soft and translucent, about 3

minutes.

Add in tofu and cook for another 4 minutes.

Add the habanero pepper, celery, mushrooms, and carrots.

Cook as you stir for 5 minutes.

Stir in the rest of the ingredients.

Simmer for 25 to 35 minutes or until cooked through.

Remove and discard the bay leaves.

Per serving: Cal 328; Fat 18g; Net Carbs 9.7g; Protein 21g

Tasty Tofu & Swiss Chard Dip

Ingredients for 4 servings

2 tbsp mayonnaise

2 cups Swiss chard

½ cup tofu, pressed, drained, crumbled

¼ cup almond milk

1 tsp nutritional yeast

1 garlic clove, minced

2 tbsp olive oil

Salt and pepper to taste

½ tsp paprika

½ tsp mint leaves, chopped

Directions and Total Time: approx. 10 minutes

Fill a pot with salted water and boil Swiss chard over medium heat for 5-6

minutes, until wilted.

Puree the remaining ingredients, except for the mayonnaise, in a food processor.

Season with salt and black pepper.

Stir in the Swiss chard and mayonnaise to get a homogeneous mixture.

Per serving: Cal 136; Fat 11g; Net Carbs 6.3g; Protein 3.1g

Roasted Cauliflower with Bell Peppers

Ingredients for 4 servings

1 lb cauliflower florets

2 bell peppers, halved

¼ cup olive oil

2 onions, quartered

Salt and black pepper, to taste

½ tsp cayenne pepper

Directions and Total Time: approx. 40 minutes

Preheat oven to 425 F.

Line a large baking sheet with parchment paper and spread out the

cauliflower, onion, and bell peppers.

Sprinkle olive oil, black pepper, salt and cayenne pepper and toss to

combine well.

Roast for 35 minutes as you toss in intervals until they start to brown.

Per serving: Cal 186; Fat 15g; Net Carbs 8.2g; Protein 3.9g

Cauliflower-Kale Dip

Ingredients for 4 servings

¼ cup olive oil

1 lb cauliflower florets

2 cups kale

Salt and black pepper, to taste

1 garlic clove, minced

1 tbsp sesame paste

1 tbsp fresh lime juice

½ tsp garam masala

Directions and Total Time: approx. 10 minutes

In a large pot filled with salted water over medium heat, steam cauliflower

until tender for 5 minutes.

Add in the kale and continue to cook for another 2-3 minutes.

Drain, transfer to a blender and pulse until smooth.

Place in garam masala, oil, black pepper, fresh lime juice, garlic, salt and

sesame paste.

Blend the mixture until well combined.

Decorate with some additional olive oil and serve.

Per serving: Cal 185; Fat 16.5g; Net Carbs 3.9g; Protein 3.5g

Zucchini Pasta with Avocado & Capers

Ingredients for 4 servings

2 tbsp olive oil

4 zucchinis, julienned or spiralized

½ cup pesto

2 avocados, sliced

¼ cup capers

¼ cup basil, chopped

¼ cup sun-dried tomatoes, chopped

Directions and Total Time: approx. 15 minutes

Cook zucchini spaghetti in half of the warm olive oil over medium heat for 4

minutes.

Transfer to a plate.

Stir in pesto, basil, salt, tomatoes, and capers.

Top with avocado slices.

Per serving: Cal 449; Fat 42g; Net Carbs 8.4g;
Protein 6.3g

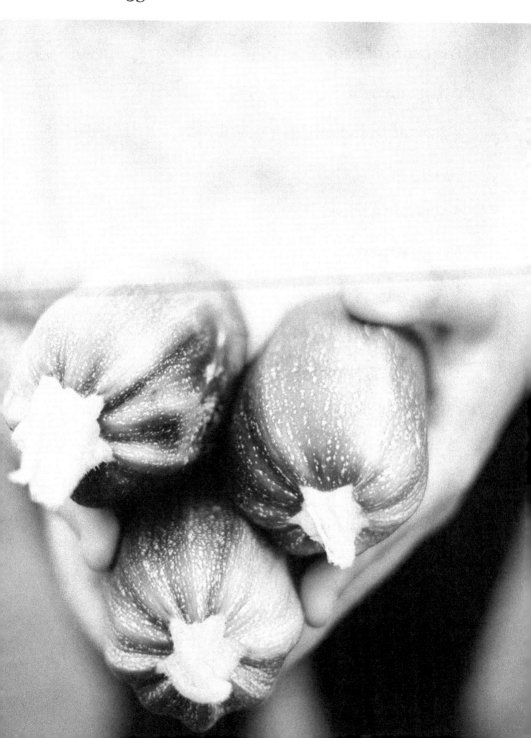

Stewed Vegetables

Ingredients for 4 servings

2 tbsp olive oil

1 shallot, chopped

1 garlic clove, minced

1 tsp paprika

1 carrot, chopped

2 tomatoes, chopped

1 head cabbage, shredded

2 cups green beans, chopped

2 bell peppers, sliced

Salt and black pepper to taste

2 tbsp parsley, chopped

1 cup vegetable broth

Directions and Total Time: approx. 32 minutes

Warm the olive oil in a saucepan over medium heat and sauté onion and

garlic to be fragrant, for 2 minutes.

Stir in bell peppers, carrot, cabbage, and green beans, paprika, salt, and

pepper, add vegetable broth and tomatoes, and cook on low heat for 25

minutes to soften.

Serve sprinkled with parsley.

Per serving: Cal 310; Fat 26.4g; Net Carbs 6g; Protein 8g

Sauteed Tofu with Pistachios

Ingredients for 4 servings

2 tbsp olive oil

8 oz firm tofu, cubed

1 tbsp tomato paste

1 tbsp balsamic vinegar

1 tsp garlic powder

1 tsp onion powder

Salt and black pepper to taste

1 cup pistachios, chopped

Directions and Total Time: approx. 15 minutes

Heat the oil in a skillet over medium heat and cook the tofu for 3 minutes

while stirring to brown.

Mix the tomato paste, garlic powder, onion powder, and vinegar; add to the

tofu.

Stir, season with salt and black pepper, and cook for another 4 minutes.

Add the pistachios.

Stir and cook on low heat for 3 minutes to be fragrant.

Per serving: Cal 335; Fat 27g; Net Carbs 6.3g; Protein 16.5g

Curried Cauliflower & Mushrooms Bake

Ingredients for 4 servings

1 head cauliflower, cut into florets

1 cup mushrooms, halved

4 garlic cloves, minced

1 red onion, sliced

2 tomatoes, chopped

¼ cup coconut oil, melted

1 tsp chili paprika paste

½ tsp curry powder

Salt and black pepper, to taste

Directions and Total Time: approx. 30 minutes

Set oven to 380 F and grease a baking dish with the coconut oil.

In a large bowl, toss the cauliflower and mushrooms, garlic, onion, tomatoes, chili paprika paste, curry, black pepper, and salt.

Spread out on the baking dish and roast for 20-25 minutes, turning once.

Place in a plate and drizzle over the cooking juices to serve.

Per serving: Cal 171; Fat 15.7g; Net Carbs 6.9g; Protein 3.5g

Roasted Tomatoes with Cheese Crust

Ingredients for 4 servings

3 tomatoes, sliced

2 tbsp olive oil

½ cup pepitas seeds

1 tbsp nutritional yeast

Salt and black pepper, to taste

1 tsp garlic puree

2 tbsp parsley. chopped

Directions and Total Time: approx. 15 minutes

Preheat oven to 380 F and grease a baking pan with olive oil.

Drizzle olive oil over the tomatoes.

In a food processor, add pepitas seeds, nutritional yeast, garlic puree, salt

and pepper, and pulse until the desired consistency is attained.

Press the mixture firmly onto each slice of tomato.

Set the tomato slices on the prepared baking pan and bake for 10 minutes.

Serve sprinkled with parsley.

Per serving: Cal 165; Fat 15g; Net Carbs 3.2g; Protein 6.2g

Coconut Milk Shake with Blackberries

Ingredients for 2 servings

½ cup water

1 ½ cups coconut milk

2 cups fresh blackberries

¼ tsp vanilla extract

1 tbsp vegan protein powder

Directions and Total Time: approx. 5 minutes

In a blender, combine all the ingredients and blend well until you attain a

uniform and creamy consistency.

Divide in glasses and serve!

Per serving: Cal 253; Fat 22g; Net Carbs 5.6g; Protein 3.3g

Spicy Cauliflower Falafel

Ingredients for 2 servings

4 tbsp olive oil

1 head cauliflower, cut into florets

1/3 cup silvered ground almonds

½ tsp ground cumin

1 tsp parsley, chopped

Salt to taste

1 tsp chili pepper

3 tbsp coconut flour

2 eggs

Directions and Total Time: approx. 15 minutes

Blitz the cauliflower in a food processor until a grain meal consistency is

formed.

Transfer to a bowl, add in the ground almonds, ground cumin, parsley, salt, chili pepper, and coconut flour, and mix until evenly combined.

Beat the eggs in a bowl and mix with the cauli mixture.

Shape ¼ cup each into patties and set aside.

Warm olive oil in a frying pan over medium heat and fry the patties for 5

minutes on each side to be firm and browned.

Remove onto a wire rack to cool, share into serving plates, and serve.

Per serving: Cal 343; Fat 31.2g; Net Carbs 3.7g; Protein 8.5g

Vegan Coconut Green Soup

Ingredients for 4 servings

1 broccoli head, chopped

1 cup spinach

1 onion, chopped

1 garlic clove, minced

½ cup leeks

3 cups vegetable stock

½ cup coconut milk

2 tbsp coconut oil

1 bay leaf

Salt and black pepper, to taste

2 tbsp coconut yogurt

Directions and Total Time: approx. 30 minutes

Warm coconut oil in a large pot over medium heat.

Add onion, leeks, and garlic and cook for 5 minutes.

Add broccoli and cook for an additional 5 minutes.

Pour in the stock over and add the bay leaf.

Close the lid, bring to a boil and reduce the heat.

Simmer for about 10 minutes.

Add spinach and cook for 3 more minutes.

Discard the bay leaf and blend the soup with a hand blender.

Stir in the coconut cream, salt and black pepper.

Divide among serving bowls and garnish with a swirl of coconut yogurt.

Per serving: Cal 272; Fat 25g; Net Carbs 4.3g; Protein 4.5g

Chocolate Nut Granola

Ingredients for 4 servings

¼ cup cocoa powder

1/3 tbsp coconut oil, melted

¼ cup almond flakes

¼ cup almond milk

¼ tbsp xylitol

1/8 tsp salt

1/3 tsp lime zest

¼ tsp ground cinnamon

¼ cup pecans, chopped

¼ cup almonds, slivered

1 tbsp pumpkin seeds

2 tbsp sunflower seeds

2 tbsp flax seed

Directions and Total Time: approx. 60 minutes

Preheat oven to 300 F and line a baking dish with parchment paper.

Set aside.

Mix almond flakes, cocoa powder, ground cinnamon, almonds, xylitol,

pumpkin seeds, sunflower seeds, flax seed, and salt in a bowl.

In a separate bowl, whisk coconut oil, almond milk and lemon zest until

combined.

Pour over the other mixture and stir to coat.

Lay the mixture in an even layer onto the baking dish.

Bake for 50 minutes, making sure that you shake gently in intervals of 15

minutes.

Let cool completely before serving.

Per serving: Cal 273; Fat 26g; Net Carbs 8.9g; Protein 4.6g

Kale with Carrot Noodles

Ingredients for 4 servings

4 tbsp olive oil

2 carrots, spiralized

¼ cup vegetable broth

1 garlic clove, minced

1 cup chopped kale

Salt and black pepper to serve

Directions and Total Time: approx. 15 minutes

Place a saucepan over low heat and pour in the vegetable broth and carrot

noodles.

Bring to a simmer for 3 minutes; strain and set aside.

Warm olive oil in a skillet and sauté garlic and kale until the kale is wilted.

Pour in carrots, season with salt and pepper, and stir-fry for 4 minutes.

Serve with grilled pork.

Per serving: Cal 341; Net Carbs 8g; Fat 28g; Protein 6g

One-Pan Curried Tofu with Cabbage

Ingredients for 4 servings

2 tbsp coconut oil

3 tbsp olive oil

2 cups extra firm tofu, cubed

½ cup grated coconut

1 tsp yellow curry powder

½ tsp onion powder

2 cups Napa cabbage

Lemon wedges for serving

Directions and Total Time: approx. 55 minutes

In a bowl, mix grated coconut, curry powder, salt, and onion powder.

Toss in tofu.

Heat coconut oil in a skillet and fry tofu until golden brown; transfer to a

plate.

In the same skillet, melt half of the olive oil and sauté the cabbage until

slightly caramelized.

Place the cabbage into plates with tofu and lemon wedges.

Drizzle the remaining olive oil over the cabbage and tofu.

Serve.

Per serving: Cal 729; Net Carbs 4g; Fat 61g; Protein 36g

DELICIOUS VEGETARIAN RECIPES (FREE EXTRA)

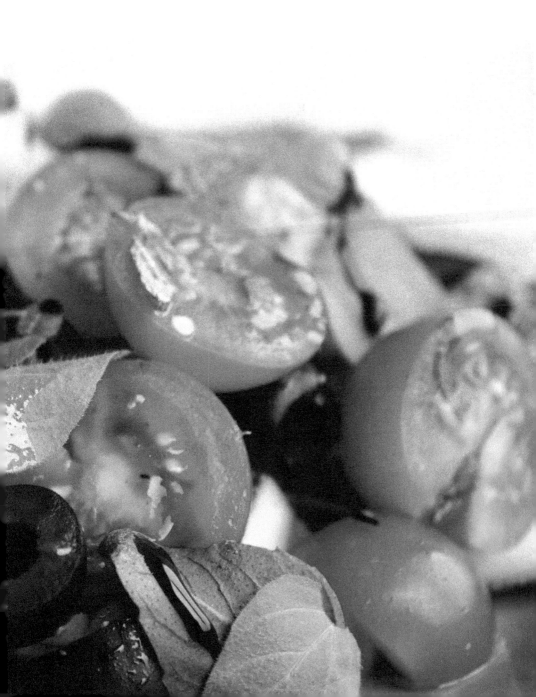

Cheesy Zucchini Muffins

Ingredients for 6 servings

1 large egg

5 tbsp olive oil

½ cup almond flour

1 tsp baking powder

½ tsp baking soda

½ cup grated cheddar cheese

1 ½ tsp mustard powder

1/3 cup almond milk

2 zucchinis, grated

6 green olives, sliced

1 spring onion, chopped

1 red bell pepper, chopped

1 tbsp freshly chopped thyme

Salt and black pepper to taste

Directions and Total Time: approx. 40 minutes

Preheat oven to 340 F.

In a bowl, combine almond flour, baking powder, baking soda, mustard

powder, salt, and pepper.

In another bowl, whisk almond milk, egg, and olive oil.

Mix the wet ingredients into dry ingredients and add cheese, zucchini,

olives, spring onion, bell pepper, and thyme; mix well.

Spoon the batter into greased muffin cups and bake for 30 minutes or until

golden brown.

Per serving: Cal 169; Net Carbs 1.6g; Fat 16g; Protein 4g

Eggplant & Tomato Gratin

Ingredients for 4 servings

1/_ cup melted butter

2 eggplants, sliced

2 garlic cloves, minced

1 red onion, sliced

7 oz tomato sauce

2 tbsp Parmesan, grated

¼ cup chopped fresh parsley

Salt and black pepper to taste

Directions and Total Time: approx. 25 minutes

Preheat oven to 400 F.

Line a baking sheet with parchment paper.

Brush eggplants with butter.

Bake until lightly browned, 20 minutes.

Heat the remaining butter in a skillet and sauté garlic and onion until

fragrant and soft, about 3 minutes.

Stir in tomato sauce and season with salt and pepper.

Simmer for 10 minutes.

Remove eggplants from the oven and spread the tomato sauce on top.

Sprinkle with Parmesan cheese and parsley and serve.

Per serving: Cal 597; Net Carbs 12g; Fat 51g; Protein 26g

Cauliflower & Pepper Gratin

Ingredients for 4 servings

1 head cauliflower, chopped

1 white onion, finely chopped

1 green bell pepper, chopped

½ cup celery stalks, chopped

2 oz butter, melted

1 cup mayonnaise

4 oz grated Parmesan

1 tsp red chili flakes

Directions and Total Time: approx. 35 minutes

Preheat oven to 400 F.

In a bowl, mix cauliflower, mayonnaise, butter, and chili flakes.

Pour the mixture into a greased baking dish and distribute the onion, celery,

and bell pepper evenly on top.

Sprinkle with Parmesan cheese and bake until golden, 20 minutes.

Serve.

Per serving: Cal 471; Net Carbs 4g; Fat 41g; Protein 36g

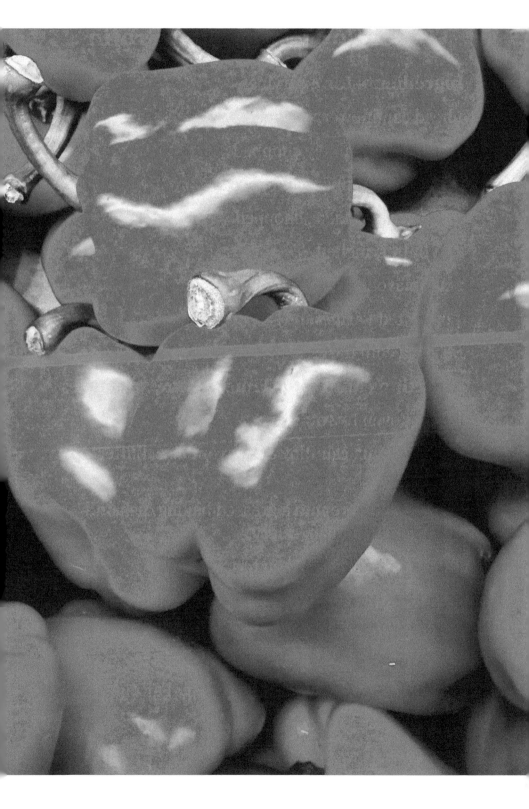

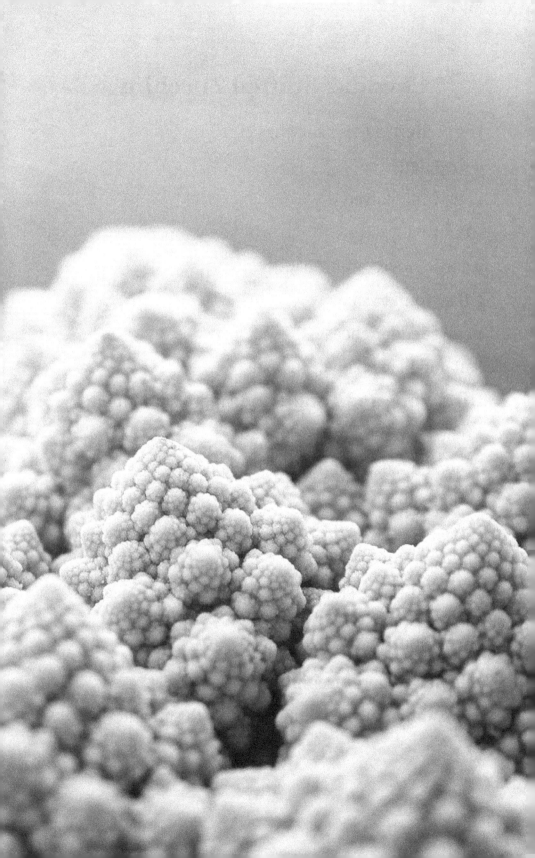

Cheddar Stuffed Zucchini

Ingredients for 2 servings

4 tbsp butter

1 zucchini, halved

1 ½ oz baby kale

2 garlic cloves, minced

2 tbsp tomato sauce

1 cup cheddar cheese

Salt and black pepper to taste

Directions and Total Time: approx. 40 minutes

Preheat oven to 375 F.

Scoop out zucchini pulp with a spoon.

Keep the flesh.

Grease a baking sheet with cooking spray and place in the zucchini boats.

Melt butter in a skillet over medium heat and sauté garlic until fragrant and

slightly browned, 4 minutes.

Add in kale and zucchini pulp.

Cook until the kale wilts; season with salt and pepper.

Spoon tomato sauce into the boats and spread to coat evenly.

Spoon kale mixture into the zucchinis and sprinkle with cheddar cheese.

Bake for 25 minutes.

Per serving: Cal 617; Net Carbs 4g; Fat 61g; Protein 19g

Butternut Squash Roast with Chimichurri

Ingredients for 4 servings

1 lb butternut squash

½ red bell pepper, chopped

1 jalapeño pepper, chopped

Zest and juice of 1 lemon

1 tbsp butter, melted

1 cup olive oil

½ cup chopped fresh parsley

2 garlic cloves, minced

3 tbsp toasted pine nuts

Salt and black pepper to taste

Directions and Total Time: approx. 15 minutes

In a bowl, add lemon zest and juice, bell pepper, jalapeño, olive oil, parsley,

garlic, salt, and pepper.

Use an immersion blender to grind the ingredients until desired consistency

is achieved; set chimichurri aside.

Slice the squash into rounds and remove the seeds.

Drizzle with butter and season with salt and pepper.

Preheat grill pan over medium heat and cook the squash for 2 minutes on

each side.

Scatter pine nuts on top and serve with chimichurri.

Per serving: Cal 647; Net Carbs 6g; Fat 44g; Protein 49g

Zucchini Pasta a la Bolognese

Ingredients for 4 servings

2 lbs zucchini, spiralized

1 carrot, chopped

½ lb ground pork

2 tbsp butter

3 oz olive oil

1 white onion, chopped

1 garlic clove, minced

2 tbsp tomato paste

1 ½ cups crushed tomatoes

1 tbsp dried basil

1 tbsp Worcestershire sauce

Salt and black pepper to taste

Directions and Total Time: approx. 45 minutes

Warm olive oil in a saucepan and sauté onion, garlic, and carrot for 3

minutes.

Pour in ground pork, tomato paste, tomatoes, salt, pepper, basil, some

water, and Worcestershire sauce.

Stir and cook for 15 minutes.

Melt butter in a skillet and toss in zoodles quickly, about 1 minute; season.

Serve the zoodles topped with the sauce.

Per serving: Cal 431; Net Carbs 6g; Fat 29g; Protein 19g

Roasted Pepper with Tofu

Ingredients for 4 servings

2 ½ cups cubed tofu

4 orange bell peppers

1 cucumber, diced

1 large tomato, chopped

3 oz cream cheese

¾ cup mayonnaise

1 tbsp melted butter

1 tsp dried parsley

1 tsp dried basil

Salt and black pepper to taste

Directions and Total Time: approx. 20 minutes

Preheat a broiler to 450 F.

Line a baking sheet with parchment paper.

In a salad bowl, combine cream cheese, mayonnaise, cucumber, tomato,

salt, pepper, and parsley; refrigerate.

Arrange bell peppers and tofu on the paper-lined baking sheet, drizzle with

melted butter, and season with basil, salt, and pepper.

Use hands to rub the ingredients until evenly coated.

Bake for 15 minutes until the peppers have charred lightly and the tofu

browned.

Per serving: Cal 838; Net Carbs 8g; Fat 81g; Protein 31g

Feta & Olive Pizza

Ingredients for 4 servings

1 tbsp olive oil

½ cup almond flour

2 tbsp ground psyllium husk

¼ tsp salt

¼ tsp red chili flakes

¼ tsp dried Greek seasoning

1 cup crumbled feta cheese

3 plum tomatoes, sliced

6 Kalamata olives, chopped

5 basil leaves, chopped

Directions and Total Time: approx. 30 minutes

Preheat oven to 390 F.

Line a baking sheet with parchment paper.

In a bowl, mix almond flour, salt, psyllium powder, olive oil, and 1 cup of

lukewarm water until dough forms.

Spread the mixture on the baking sheet and bake for 10 minutes.

Sprinkle the red chili flakes and Greek seasoning on the crust and top with the feta cheese.

Arrange the tomatoes and olives on top.

Bake for 10 minutes.

Garnish the pizza with basil, slice, and serve warm.

Per serving: Cal 281; Net Carbs 4.5g; Fats 12g; Protein 8g

Chargrilled Zucchini withAvocado Pesto

Ingredients for 4 servings

1 avocado, chopped

3 oz spinach, chopped

2 zucchinis, sliced

¾ cup olive oil

2 tbsp melted butter

2 oz pecans

1 garlic clove, minced

Juice of 1 lemon

Salt and black pepper to taste

Directions and Total Time: approx. 20 minutes

Put the spinach in a food processor along with avocado, half of lemon juice,

garlic, olive oil, and pecans and blend until smooth; season with salt and

pepper.

Pour the pesto into a bowl and set aside.

Season zucchini with the remaining lemon juice, salt, pepper, and butter.

Preheat a grill pan and cook the zucchini slices until browned.

Remove to a plate, spoon the pesto to the side, and serve.

Per serving: Cal 548; Net Carbs 6g; Fat 46g; Protein 25g

Coconut Avocado Tart

Ingredients for 4 servings

1¼ cups grated Parmesan

½ cup cream cheese

1 egg

4 tbsp coconut flour

4 tbsp chia seeds

¾ cup almond flour

1 tbsp psyllium husk powder

1 tsp baking powder

3 tbsp coconut oil

2 ripe avocados, chopped

1 cup mayonnaise

1 jalapeño pepper, chopped

½ tsp onion powder

2 tbsp fresh parsley, chopped

Directions and Total Time: approx. 80 minutes

Preheat oven to 350 F.

In a food processor, add coconut flour, chia seeds, almond flour, psyllium

husk, baking powder, coconut oil, and 4 tbsp water.

Blend until the resulting dough forms into a ball.

Line a springform pan with parchment paper and spread the dough.

Bake for 15 minutes.

In a bowl, put avocado, mayonnaise, egg, parsley, jalapeño pepper, onion

powder, cream cheese, and Parmesan cheese; mix well.

Remove the piecrust when ready and fill with the creamy mixture.

Bake for 35 minutes until lightly golden brown.

Per serving: Cal 891; Net Carbs 10g; Fat 71g; Protein 24g

Baked Veggies with Green Salad

Ingredients for 2 servings

½ zucchini, sliced

¹⁄_ eggplant, sliced

¼ cup coconut oil

2 tbsp pecans

Juice of ½ lemon

5 oz cheddar cheese, cubed

10 Kalamata olives

1 oz mixed salad greens

½ cup mayonnaise

½ tsp Cayenne pepper

Directions and Total Time: approx. 35 minutes

Line a baking sheet with parchment paper.

Arrange zucchini and eggplant slices on the sheet.

Brush with coconut oil and sprinkle with cayenne pepper.

Set the oven to broil and l broil the vegetables until golden brown, about 18

minutes.

Remove to a serving platter and drizzle with lemon juice.

Arrange cheddar cheese, olives, pecans, and mixed greens next to baked

veggies.

Top with mayonnaise and serve.

Per serving: Cal 509g; Net Carbs 8g; Fat 31g; Protein 22g

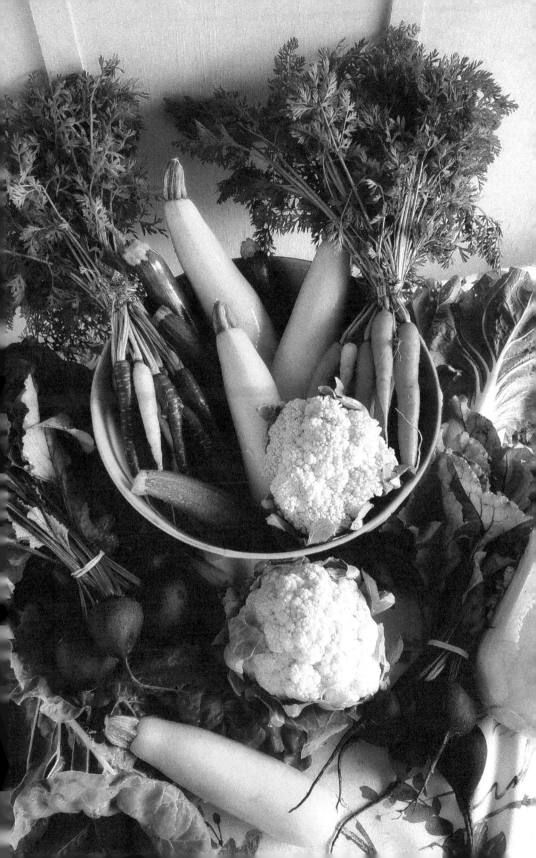

Hot Broccoli Rabe

Ingredients for 4 servings

1 tbsp olive oil

1 tbsp melted butter

3 cups broccoli rabe, chopped

1 orange bell pepper, sliced

1 garlic clove, minced

1 tbsp red chili flakes

Salt and black pepper to taste

Directions and Total Time: approx. 15 minutes

Blanch broccoli in lightly salted water for 3 minutes or until softened; drain.

Heat butter and olive oil in a skillet over medium heat and sauté garlic and

bell pepper until softened, 5 minutes.

Toss in broccoli.

Sprinkle with flakes.

Per serving: Cal 72; Net Carbs 1.2g; Fat 6.4g; Protein 1.2g

Walnut & Feta Loaf

Ingredients for 4 servings

1 green bell pepper, chopped

1 red bell pepper, chopped

2 white onions, chopped

4 garlic cloves, minced

1 lb feta, cubed

3 tbsp olive oil

2 tbsp soy sauce

¾ cup chopped walnuts

Salt and black pepper

1 tbsp Italian mixed herbs

½ tsp swerve sugar

¼ cup golden flaxseed meal

1 tbsp sesame seeds

½ cup tomato sauce

Directions and Total Time: approx. 70 minutes

Preheat oven to 350 F.

In a bowl, combine olive oil, onion, garlic, feta, soy sauce, walnuts, salt, pepper, Italian herbs, swerve sugar, golden flaxseed meal and mix with

your hands.

Pour the mixture into a bowl and stir in sesame seeds and bell peppers.

Transfer the mixture into a greased loaf and spoon tomato sauce on top.

Bake for 45 minutes.

Turn onto a chopping board, slice, and serve.

Per serving: Cal 429; Net Carbs 2.5g; Fat 28g; Protein 24g

Delicious Mushroom Pie

Ingredients for 4 servings

For the piecrust

4 whole eggs

¼ cup butter, cold and crumbled

¼ cup almond flour

3 tbsp coconut flour

3 tbsp erythritol

1 ½ tsp vanilla extract

½ tsp salt

For the filling

2 cups mixed mushrooms, chopped

1 cup green beans, cut into 3 pieces each

2 eggs, lightly beaten

2 tbsp butter

1 yellow onion, chopped

2 garlic cloves, minced

1 green bell pepper, diced

¼ cup heavy cream

1/3 cup sour cream

½ cup almond milk

¼ tsp nutmeg powder

1 tbsp chopped parsley

1 cup grated Monterey Jack

Salt and black pepper to taste

Directions and Total Time: approx. 2 hours

Preheat oven to 350 F.

In a bowl, mix almond and coconut flours, and salt.

Add in butter and mix until crumbly.

Stir in erythritol and vanilla extract.

Pour in the eggs one after another while mixing until formed into a ball.

Flatten the dough on a clean flat surface, cover with plastic wrap, and

refrigerate for 1 hour.

Dust a clean flat surface with almond flour, unwrap the dough and roll out

into a large rectangle.

Fit into a greased pie pan and with a fork, prick the base of the crust.

Bake for 15 minutes; let cool.

For the filling, melt butter in a skillet over medium heat and sauté onion and

garlic for 3 minutes.

Add in mushrooms, bell pepper, and green beans; cook for 5 minutes.

In a bowl, beat heavy cream, sour cream, almond milk, and eggs.

Season with salt, pepper, and nutmeg.

Stir in parsley and cheese.

Spread the mushroom mixture on the baked pastry and spread the cheese

filling on top.

Place the pie in the oven and bake for 35 minutes.

Slice and serve.

Per serving: Cal 531; Net Carbs 6.5g; Fat 39g; Protein 21g

Vegetable Biryani

Ingredients for 4 servings

2 tbsp olive oil

3 tbsp ghee

1 cup sliced cremini mushrooms

6 cups cauli rice

3 white onions, chopped

6 garlic cloves, minced

1 tsp ginger puree

1 tbsp turmeric powder

2 cups chopped tomatoes

1 habanero pepper, minced

1 tbsp tomato puree

1 cup diced paneer cheese

½ cup spinach, chopped

½ cup kale, chopped

¼ cup chopped parsley

1 cup Greek yogurt

Salt and black pepper to taste

Directions and Total Time: approx. 1 hour 20 minutes

Preheat oven to 400 F.

Microwave cauli rice for 1 minute.

Remove and season with salt and black pepper; set aside.Melt ghee in a

pan over medium heat and sauté onions, garlic, ginger puree, and turmeric.

Cook for 15 minutes, stirring regularly.

Add in tomatoes, habanero pepper, and tomato puree; cook for 5 minutes.

Stir in mushrooms, paneer cheese, spinach, kale, and 1/3 cup water and

simmer for 15 minutes or until the mushrooms soften.

Turn the heat off and stir in yogurt.

Spoon half of the stew into a bowl.

Sprinkle half of the parsley over the stew in the pan, half of the cauli rice,

and dust with turmeric.

Repeat the layering a second time including the reserved stew.

Drizzle with olive oil and bake for 25 minutes.

Serve.

Per serving: Cal 351; Net Carbs 2g; Fat 19g; Protein 16g

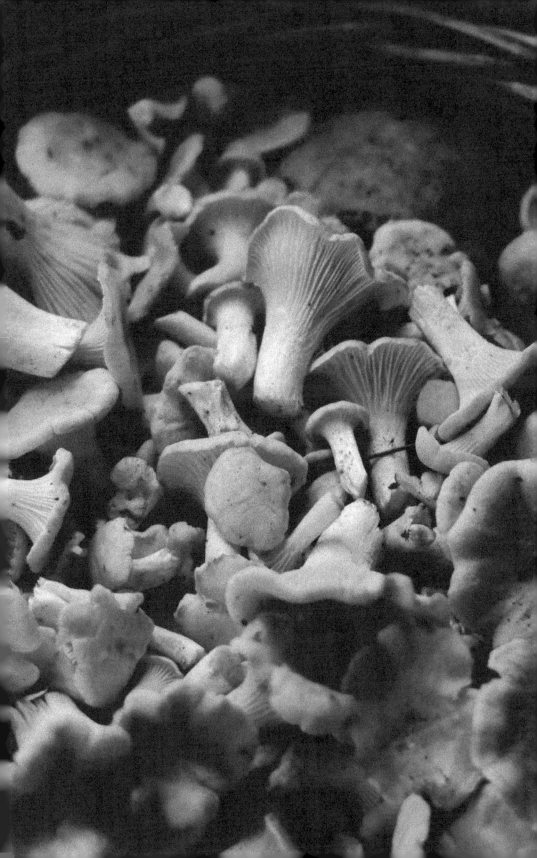

Charred Broccoli with Tamarind Sauce

Ingredients for 6 servings

4 tbsp melted butter

½ cup peanut butter

1 white onion, finely chopped

1 head broccoli, cut into florets

1 small red chili, chopped

1 garlic clove, peeled

1-inch ginger, peeled

2 tbsp tamarind sauce

1 tsp swerve brown sugar

1 tsp garlic powder

1 tsp dried basil

3 tbsp parsley, chopped

½ lemon, juiced

Salt and black pepper to taste

Directions and Total Time: approx. 30 minutes

Bring to a boil 2 cups of water in a pot and blanch broccoli for 2 minutes;

drain.

In a bowl, mix butter, onion, garlic powder, basil, salt, pepper.

Toss broccoli in the mixture and marinate for 5 minutes.

Heat a grill pan over high and cook broccoli until charred, turning once.

Transfer to a plate.

Place garlic and ginger in a blender and pulse until broken into pieces.

Add in lemon juice, peanut butter, tamarind sauce, brown sugar, parsley,

chili, and 1/3 cup water.

Blend until smooth.

Top the broccoli with the sauce.

Per serving: Cal 271; Net Carbs 5g; Fat 18g; Protein 7.6g

Zucchini & Cheese Casserole

Ingredients for 4 servings

2 tbsp olive oil

3 tbsp salted butter, melted

3 large zucchinis, sliced

¼ cup grated mozzarella

2/3 cup grated Parmesan

1 garlic clove, minced

1 tsp dried thyme

Directions and Total Time: approx. 25 minutes

Preheat oven to 350 F.

Pour zucchini in a bowl; add in butter, olive oil, garlic, and thyme; toss to

coat.

Spread onto a baking dish and sprinkle with the mozzarella and Parmesan

cheeses.

Bake for 15 minutes.

Serve warm.

Per serving: Cal 202; Net Carbs 3g; Fat 16g; Protein 7.4g

Crispy Avocado with Parmesan Sauce

Ingredients for 4 servings

2 tbsp olive oil

3 tbsp almond flour

1 ½ cups almond milk

5 tbsp melted butter

1 cup grated cheddar cheese

4 oz cream cheese, softened

¼ cup grated Parmesan

2 avocados, sliced

¼ tsp mustard powder

¼ tsp garlic powder

2 tbsp sriracha sauce

Black pepper to taste

Directions and Total Time: approx. 16 minutes

Whisk 3 tbsps of butter with almond flour in a saucepan and cook until

golden.

Whisk in almond milk, mustard powder, garlic, and black pepper.

Cook, whisking continuously until thickened, 2 minutes.

Stir in the cheeses until they are melted; set aside.

In a bowl, toss avocado in remaining butter and sriracha sauce.

Heat olive oil in a pan and cook avocado until golden, turning halfway, 4

minutes in total.

Plate and pour the cheese sauce all over to serve.

Per serving: Cal 551; Net Carbs 3.2g; Fat 51g; Protein 10g

Green Sauté with Pine Nuts

Ingredients for 4 servings

1 tbsp olive oil

2 tbsp butter

2 heads large broccoli, riced

2 shallots, finely sliced

2 tbsp pine nuts

1 tsp swerve sugar

2 tbsp red wine vinegar

1 tsp cumin powder

1 garlic clove, minced

4 tbsp chopped parsley

Directions and Total Time: approx. 25 minutes

In a bowl, whisk shallots, swerve sugar, and vinegar and set aside.

Melt butter in a skillet and stir in cumin and garlic for 1 minute.

Add in asparagus to soften for 5 minutes.

Mix in mixed greens.

Reduce the heat to low and steam the vegetables for 1 minute.

Stir in parsley.

Drizzle with olive oil and garnish with pine nuts to serve.

Per serving: Cal 81; Net Carbs 3.5g; Fat 6.1g; Protein 1.9g

Mushrooms with Broccoli Noddles

Ingredients for 4 servings

4 large broccoli

1 cup cremini mushrooms, sliced

1 cup grated Gruyere cheese

2 tbsp olive oil

4 scallions, chopped

2 garlic cloves, minced

2 tbsp almond flour

1 ½ cups almond milk

¼ cup chopped fresh parsley

Salt and black pepper to taste

Directions and Total Time: approx. 20 minutes

Cut off the florets of the broccoli heads, leaving only the stems.

Cut the ends of the stem flatly and evenly.

Run the stems through a spiralizer to make the noodles.

Heat olive oil in a skillet and sauté the broccoli noodles, mushrooms, garlic,

and scallions until softened, 5 minutes.

In a bowl, combine almond flour and almond milk and pour the mixture over

the vegetables.

Stir and allow thickening for 2-3 minutes.

Whisk in half of the Gruyere cheese to melt and adjust the taste with salt

and black pepper.

Garnish with the remaining Gruyere cheese and parsley and serve.

Per serving: Cal 219; Net Carbs 1.4g; Fats 15g; Protein 10g

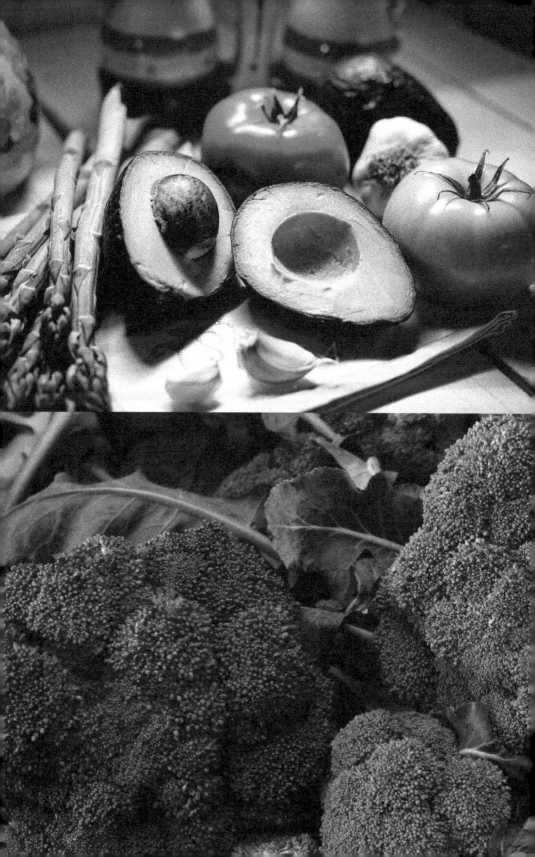

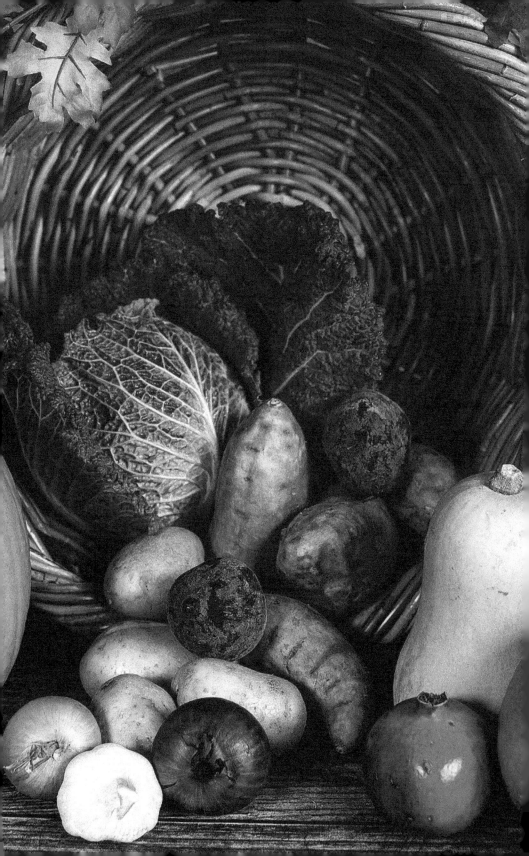

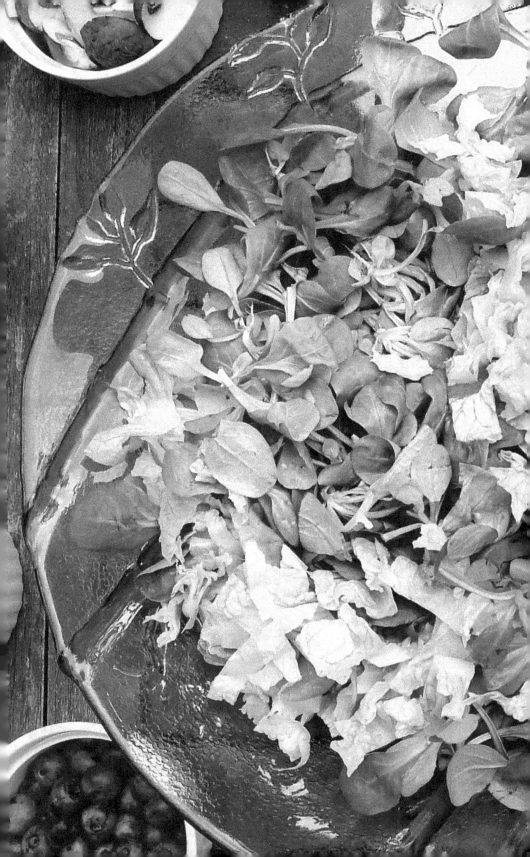

CPSIA information can be obtained
at www.ICGtesting.com
Printed in the USA
LVHW050319190421
684849LV00015B/892